M000158377

"As a therapist who aims to provide the bes[...] encourage them to purchase this journal to [...] can continue reflecting on the work we do [...] in a facilitated manner. The writing prompts provided in this journal will help clients develop greater insight into their behavior and see sustained changes over time."

—Krystle Martin, clinical and forensic psychologist, dialectical behavior therapy (DBT) trainer and consultant, clinic director at Dr. Krystle Martin & Associates, and associate graduate faculty member at Ontario Tech University

"A simple and effective daily ritual to help bring our skills to the forefront of our attention, with intention. These daily reflections offer a structured reminder to mindfully engage with the world and ourselves while reinforcing our use of the DBT skills we have learned."

—Darrell Gonzales, MSW, DBT-Linehan Board of Certification, Certified ClinicianTM; Broadleaf Health

"A missing link in the life of DBT-ers! This journal is a must-have for individuals looking to truly practice DBT in their everyday lives. As a DBT therapist and lifelong enthusiast of the practice, I know that DBT is not something that one can simply apply to one area of their life. DBT is life-changing work, and for that reason it needs to be embedded into every aspect of life. This workbook will help individuals looking to do just that."

—Shaelene Lauriano Kite, LPC, DBT-LBC, RYT, owner of DBT of South Jersey, owner of Rebelmente Training & Consulting, and host of the T-Talk Podcast

"The DBT Skills Daily Journal not only provides a brief skills tool kit at your fingertips, it delivers the format necessary to build a habit of self-reflection and mindfulness through daily journaling. This combination is sure to benefit anyone wishing for more insight into their emotional experience."

—Amanda A. Uliaszek, PhD, CPsych, associate professor of psychology at the University of Toronto

"Zambrano has developed a thoughtful and practical journal for those leaning on DBT to navigate through life's challenges and to build their life worth living. The simplicity of the practices and opportunities for reflection in *The DBT Skills Daily Journal* are a wonderful tool to support mindful skills practice in the situations where the skills are needed. I look forward to recommending this self-help tool to my clients!"

—Megan Cameron, MSW, RSW, DBT therapist in private practice, and mental health care leader

"Anyone and everyone can benefit from living life more skillfully, and this journal will help you do just that. *The DBT Skills Daily Journal* is an invaluable resource for DBT novices and veterans alike. The simple yet thought-provoking journaling prompts serve as a friendly guide helping you navigate mindfully throughout your day. Whether you are a longtime journaler or entirely new to the process, this book is for you."

—Hailey Goldberg, MSW, RSW, DBT-Linehan Board of Certification, Certified Clinician™; and founder and DBT Skills Trainer at DBT HOUSE

"'Learning' is embodying skills, acting on skills, and making skills alive in your life. May you take this book as a companion on your skill-learning journey. May you spill coffee on it, scribble all over it, bend it when pulling it out of your purse or backpack. USE IT as a prompt, a record, an encourager of your efforts to build a Life Worth Living!"

—Andrew Ekblad, PhD, CPsych, founder and director of Broadleaf Health, a DBT-Linehan Board-Certified Program

New Harbinger Journals for Change

Research shows that journaling has a universally positive effect on mental health. But in the midst of life's difficulties—such as stress, anxiety, depression, relationship problems, parenting challenges, or even obsessive or negative thoughts—where do you begin? New Harbinger *Journals for Change* combine evidence-based psychology with proven-effective guided journaling techniques to help you make lasting personal change—one page at a time. Written by renowned mental health and wellness experts, *Journals for Change* provide a creative and safe space to process difficult emotions, work through challenges, reflect on what matters, and set intentions for the future.

Since 1973, New Harbinger has published practical, user-friendly self-help books and workbooks to help readers make positive change. Our *Journals for Change* offer the same powerfully effective tools—without ever *feeling* like therapy. If you're committed to improving your mental health, these easy-to-use guided journals can help you take small, actionable steps toward lasting well-being.

For a complete list of journals in our *Journals for Change* series, visit newharbinger.com.

The DBT Skills Daily Journal

10 Minutes a Day to Soothe Your Emotions with Dialectical Behavior Therapy

DYLAN ZAMBRANO, MSW

New Harbinger Publications, Inc.

Publisher's Note

This publication is designed to provide accurate and authoritative information in regard to the subject matter covered. It is sold with the understanding that the publisher is not engaged in rendering psychological, financial, legal, or other professional services. If expert assistance or counseling is needed, the services of a competent professional should be sought.

NEW HARBINGER PUBLICATIONS is a registered trademark of New Harbinger Publications, Inc.

New Harbinger Publications is an employee-owned company.

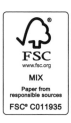

Copyright © 2023 by Dylan Zambrano
New Harbinger Publications, Inc.
5720 Shattuck Avenue
Oakland, CA 94609
www.newharbinger.com

All Rights Reserved

Cover and interior design by Amy Daniel

Acquired by Ryan Buresh

Edited by Joyce Wu

Library of Congress Cataloging-in-Publication Data on file

Printed in the United States of America

25   24   23

10   9   8   7   6   5   4   3   2   1   First Printing

Contents

Foreword

By Sheri Van Dijk, MSW, RSW

Over the years research has demonstrated the efficacy of dialectical behavior therapy, or DBT (originally created to treat borderline personality disorder), in helping people manage general emotion dysregulation more effectively, regardless of the cause. I have spent most of my career trying to make DBT more accessible to clients (and clinicians!), having seen how helpful the skills can be for a broad range of mental health problems, as well as for the more basic difficulties that will arise for most of us in life—managing stress, grief, sadness, disappointment, anger, hurt, and so on.

As a behavioral therapy, DBT emphasizes the importance of making behavioral changes specifically through monitoring your emotions, thoughts, and behaviors. This journal, created by Dylan Zambrano, will provide you with tools to engage in this important step of making changes: first, providing an overview of the skills so you can review—or learn—them, then combining this with daily prompts to help you practice the skills so that you'll be able to more fully embrace them.

Whether you find yourself struggling with intense, volatile emotions that lead to unhealthy behaviors and chaos in your life on a regular basis, or you'd simply like to improve your ability to manage emotions in healthier ways, Zambrano's *DBT Skills Daily Journal* is a wonderful tool that will aid you in your journey of making changes.

Introduction

If you've opened this journal, perhaps you've been introduced to Dialectical Behavior Therapy (DBT) before, or maybe it has been recommended to you by a healthcare provider or family member. Either way, you're in the right place. DBT was initially designed for those with challenges in regulating intense, volatile emotions and interpersonal struggles (Linehan 1993). However, emotions and relationships are at the core of human experience, which is why DBT has something to offer for all of us. So, this journal is for everyone, from beginners learning DBT coping skills for the first time to those with advanced practice.

Essential to DBT, unlike other therapy modalities, is skills training. These coping skills—which pertain to mindfulness, distress tolerance, emotion regulation, and interpersonal effectiveness—teach new ways of being and behaving to live happier, more fulfilling and balanced lives (Linehan 2014). DBT offers skills that help us to step back when we just can't stop worrying about that upcoming interview, exam, or social outing; to persevere even after a really difficult day; and to accept and move forward from loss or major life changes. Simply put, DBT skills have proven versatility and have the capacity to make us better versions of ourselves.

Ultimately, DBT skills help us respond more effectively to our emotions and within our relationships with others. To respond *effectively* means to act with intention, in a way that supports our short- *and* long-term goals and is congruent with our values.

It takes more than just knowing the skills to live your life in this way. To master these skills, you'll need to practice them regularly. And you'll need to do this during the pleasant and unpleasant moments, the simple and difficult times. In this way,

DBT skills are much like other skills—like cooking, art, or athletics—which require repeated practice to build and maintain your competency. If you stop using these skills, they become less accessible to you, and you might default to the problematic and reactive behaviors that emotions can sometimes encourage.

While coping with emotions may come naturally to some people, no one is perfect. Everyone has moments when they say or do something unhelpful when strong emotions surface. But with deliberate practice of DBT skills, you too can become more effective in how you respond to your emotions, stressful events, and conflicts with others. And in this book, the main method for deliberate practice and reflection is journaling.

Journaling helps us sort out the clutter of thoughts that we can often hold in our minds. It allows us to mindfully process information in a way that promotes reflection and intention in how we want to go about our lives.

Journaling has become a widely used practice to improve resilience to emotions like anxiety and depressive symptoms (Smyth et al. 2018); to increase optimism (Emmons and McCullough 2003) and happiness (Seligman et al. 2005); to expand our gratitude for the little things in life; and to set goals for the future.

Each prompt in this journal has been carefully designed to help you use journaling to strengthen your practice of DBT skills. At the same time, this book is not intended to be a substitute for professional advice or mental health therapy. You might find you need further education, modeling, and coaching from a trained healthcare professional to really understand DBT skills and integrate them into your life, and that's fine.

Ultimately, the hope is that with just ten minutes of journaling a day, you can begin to live a happier, healthier, and more skillful life! And you can discover your inner wisdom to help you navigate challenges, even in the most difficult moments life can bring.

First, let's review some of the DBT skills you'll reflect on and put into practice.

THE DBT SKILLS

There are four categories of DBT skills:

1. **MINDFULNESS** —the capacity to bring an open awareness to internal and external experiences that occur in the present moment

2. **DISTRESS TOLERANCE** —the ability to tolerate the inevitable pain that's experienced in life and to shift the body's emotional response to painful events when you need to, so you can find peace and return to a more grounded, manageable emotional state

3. **EMOTION REGULATION** —the capacity to understand your own emotions, decrease the frequency and intensity of unpleasant emotions, and increase your resilience and the experience of pleasant emotions

4. **INTERPERSONAL EFFECTIVENESS** —the ability to interact and communicate effectively, and engage with others in a way that maintains your relationships and self-respect

Each of these categories of DBT skills also has a subset of skills, summarized on the following pages for your reference as you navigate this journal. They'll guide your integration of the skills in your written reflections.

MINDFULNESS skills involve:

- **MINDFULLY ATTENDING:** Experience each moment just as it is, through the five senses, rather than what we think it is, through the stories we tend to tell ourselves and can assume are true. **(Skill: Observe)**

- **NONJUDGMENTAL LABELING:** Objectively labeling what we experience in the moment can help us avoid strong emotional reactions. For example, *She hasn't responded to my message since I texted her yesterday* is a neutral description of what's happening, not an assumption of what she's thinking, like *She must not like me or want to be my friend*. **(Skill: Describe, Nonjudgmentally)**

- **FULLY IMMERSING:** Engage yourself wholly in what you're experiencing in the moment. Focusing on the moment and letting go of judgments—like worries about what others are thinking about you—can allow you to be totally absorbed in what you're doing. **(Skill: Participate)**

- **INNER WISDOM:** Integrating *emotions* (what you feel) and *logic* (what you think), rather than over-relying on one and underutilizing the other, will allow you to enter a space of *wisdom* (what you know to be most effective). **(Skill: Wise Mind)**

- **COMPASSION FOR ONESELF AND OTHERS:** Pair your concern for someone's suffering—whether your own or others'—with wishes or actions to alleviate that suffering. **(Skill: Loving-Kindness)**

DISTRESS TOLERANCE skills include:

- **COLD TEMPERATURE:** Our heart rate and breath slow down when we apply cold water to the surface of the skin, primarily on the face. You can use this calming reflex to short-circuit acute emotional responses and disrupt repetitive negative thinking by orienting your attention to the immediate cold sensations. **(Skill: Tip the Temperature)**

- **REGULATED BREATHING:** Strong emotions can sometimes cause shallow breathing, raising your stress levels. By intentionally altering the breath—with deep inhales, brief holds, and extended exhales— you can tap into your innate ability for self-regulation and bring yourself to a more relaxed state when you need to. **(Skill: Paced Breathing)**

- **VIGOROUS EXERCISE:** Exercise can be another way to regulate the body's intense physical response to emotions. It doesn't have to be lengthy; brief bouts of intense exercise will work, and in a variety of forms: jumping jacks, jogging around the block, rapidly cleaning your home, and so on. **(Skill: Intense Exercise)**

- **DISTRACTION:** Distracting yourself—temporarily, of course, not in a way that becomes a means of avoiding problems—can also be helpful when you're having especially intense emotions and racing thoughts. You can use activities that occupy your attention (like puzzles, counting, or singing), generate different emotions (like listening to a joyful music playlist or watching a cute animal video), or focus on the well-being of others (like sending someone a kind message or taking care of your pets). **(Skill: Distracting)**

- **SOOTHING THE SENSES:** Use your senses—touch, taste, hearing, sight, or smell—to soothe discomfort and find ease in a difficult moment. You can listen to nature sounds, feel a fuzzy blanket, or watch the clouds float by. **(Skill: Self-Soothing)**

- **TAKING A MENTAL BREAK:** When you can't escape a stressor and must continue facing it, you can use your thoughts to make the moment more tolerable by visualizing yourself in a calming place, recalling moments of resilience in the past, or finding meaning or something to be grateful for in the difficult situation you're in. **(Skill: Improving the Moment)**

- **ACCEPTING YOUR CIRCUMSTANCES:** Much of our distress can stem from difficulty accepting the present. We might wish that things were different, fixate on what's undesirable, or believe the future will never be better. When we recognize that this is happening, we can instead resist the urge to fight with the circumstances, embrace difficult moments, and allow ourselves to experience situations and the emotions that come with them. **(Skill: Radical Acceptance)**

One important note before we proceed: some distress tolerance skills rely on rapidly altering your physiological response (e.g., your heart rate). Please consult a medical professional if you're concerned about the suitability of these skills.

Skills for **EMOTION REGULATION** include:

- **BALANCED THINKING:** The way we interpret events, which can influence how we respond to them, isn't always accurate. If you can notice your interpretations and adjust them to accurately reflect the facts of a situation, your emotions and actions can become appropriate responses to what's actually happening—not what you *think* is happening. **(Skill: Check the Facts)**

- **DOING THE OPPOSITE OF EMOTIONAL URGES:** Sometimes our emotions drive us to act in particular ways. Engaging in emotional urges isn't always the best option. Sometimes, doing the *opposite* of the urge is more effective. For instance, anger might lead to an urge to express aggression. But doing the opposite—acting kindly, or temporarily avoiding the situation until you're calm—might be more useful. **(Skill: Opposite Action)**

- **PROBLEM SOLVING TO CHANGE EMOTIONS:** Sometimes, it's not the interpretation of the circumstances that's the problem; the circumstances *are* the problem. In those moments, we can change our circumstances to change our emotions. For instance, when you're panicked because your car won't start, making alternative arrangements to get to your destination, adjusting your plans, or creating a plan to get the car fixed are actions that can solve aspects of the problem to reduce the panic. **(Skill: Problem Solving)**

- **ANTICIPATORY COPING:** We can plan out ways to cope with stressful or unfamiliar situations ahead of time when we know they're coming. **(Skill: Cope Ahead)**

- ***TREATING PHYSICAL HEALTH:*** There is a link between the body and the mind that shouldn't be overlooked. Intense, long-lasting emotions and negative moods are more likely to occur when you neglect your physical health needs. By taking care of your physical health, you can ultimately improve your mental and emotional stability. **(Skill: PLEASE)**

- ***INCREASING PLEASANT EMOTIONS:*** While many DBT skills are intended to reduce unpleasant emotions, working to increase the pleasant emotions we feel—by mindfully engaging in pleasant activities, living in accordance with our values, and doing things that are challenging and rewarding—is important too. **(Skill: Accumulating Positive Emotions & Build Mastery)**

And finally, skills for **INTERPERSONAL EFFECTIVENESS** include:

- ***RELATIONSHIP GOAL SETTING:*** When you mindfully reflect on goals you have for a relationship or a conversation before you enter it, you can better balance your needs with others' needs while preserving the relationship and your own self-respect. **(Skill: Clarifying Goals in Interpersonal Situations)**

- ***ASSERTIVE COMMUNICATION:*** Verbalize your needs to others in a calm, direct, and respectful way—one that's not aggressive or passive. **(Skill: DEAR MAN)**

- ***FOSTERING CONNECTION:*** Use respectful and likable communication that helps you achieve your objectives *and* strengthen your connections, interactions, and long-term relationships. **(Skill: GIVE)**

- **VALIDATING YOURSELF AND OTHERS:** Recognize what is valid about your or others' experiences. It doesn't mean you agree with the experience someone is having—just that you acknowledge what they or you feel ("I can see why this situation would make you feel upset"; "It's okay that I feel this anxious"). **(Skill: Validation)**

- **NOURISHING YOUR SELF-RESPECT:** It's important to confidently stand up for yourself, your beliefs, and your values (without apologizing, assuming you're wrong or undeserving, or demanding you always get your way). **(Skill: FAST)**

Each day of this journal features recurring prompts to help you attend to your emotions, set intentions for how you'll be skillful in the day to come, and reassess your experience at the day's end (the ways in which you were effective, and the DBT skills you practiced). And each day you complete the journal, you'll also encounter a prompt to help you practice the DBT skills you just read about and reflect on how you'll integrate your insights to guide your actions in your everyday life. With the use of these simple, practical, and powerful coping skills, you can learn to behave in ways that help you live a fulfilling life—without strong feelings or tough circumstances running the show. This daily journal will help you start.

Let's dive in.

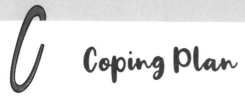

Coping Plan

Complete this individualized coping plan to help you prepare ahead of time for emotionally overwhelming and challenging moments. Refer to this page as needed.

MY TRIGGERS:

○ _____

_____

○ _____

_____

○ _____

_____

THE WARNING SIGNS:

_____

_____

_____

_____

_____

_____

ACTIVITIES I FIND SOOTHING AND CALMING:

_____

_____

_____

_____

_____

You'll also find a printable version at http://www.newharbinger.com/51963, if you'd like to print it out and post it somewhere handy.

THINGS I CAN DO TO DISTRACT MYSELF:

- ☐ _____
- ☐ _____
- ☐ _____
- ☐ _____
- ☐ _____
- ☐ _____
- ☐ _____

REASONS AND MOTIVATIONS TO GET THROUGH DIFFICULT MOMENTS:

_____
_____
_____
_____
_____
_____
_____

SELF-ENCOURAGING AND COMPASSIONATE STATEMENTS:

_____
_____
_____
_____
_____

IF IT IS AN EMERGENCY, CALL A LOCAL EMERGENCY SERVICE OR CRISIS LINE, OR VISIT YOUR NEAREST EMERGENCY ROOM

PEOPLE I CAN CALL FOR SUPPORT:

- ☐ _____
- ☐ _____
- ☐ _____

··· Skills Coach ···

When you're going through a difficult moment, the following prompts can coach you through your options for problem solving and coping. This is not intended to replace proper therapeutic advice or treat all problems, but to guide your decision-making when you're attempting to soothe your emotions and find a resolution.

1. Label your emotion and its intensity:

Emotion: _____

Mild				Moderate					Severe
1	2	3	4	5	6	7	8	9	10

2. Before reacting on your emotions:

- Pause and temporarily remove yourself from the situation.
- Notice what is happening around you and within you.
- Consider if your emotions are encouraging behaviors that are effective.

3. Consider your health factors. Do you need to...

- Eat something?
- Take your prescribed medications?
- Take care of any physical health needs or pain?
- Engage in physical activity or exercise?
- Catch up on sleep?
- Do some self-care?

4. If you're in the moderate to severe range, try a few of the following:

- Cold temperature: splash cold water on your face, take a cold shower, hold an ice pack.

- Regulated breathing: take some deep breaths with extended exhales.

- Distraction: watch videos, read, cook, clean or organize, talk to someone, do work, play a game.

- Soothe the senses: listen to pleasant music, sip a hot beverage, take a warm bath, cuddle with a pet, walk in nature.

- Vigorous exercise: a fast-paced walk, jumping jacks, and so forth.

5. After your emotions have settled, ask yourself: *Is there a problem remaining to be solved?* If yes:

- Consider what the problem is and what your goals are right now.

- Consider what needs to be done to change or resolve the problem, and put this into action.

6. If the problem cannot be resolved:

- Embrace the circumstances with acceptance.

- Adopt a relaxing posture and take actions to soothe uncomfortable emotions.

- Express supportive words to yourself or do something kind for yourself.

- Find meaning or positive aspects in the difficult experience.

You can also find an extended, printable copy of the Skills Coach at
http://www.newharbinger.com/51963.

Intention Setting

The act of setting intentions is about being purposeful in how you live your life each day. Without intentions, you leave the day up to chance, without a clear direction or commitment to what you wish to accomplish. Use the prompts below to set your intentions for your journaling practice before you begin.

How often and when do I wish to journal?

_____

_____

Why is this important to me? What do I hope to gain, accomplish, or change?

_____

_____

What obstacles might arise?

_____

_____

What skills or strategies will help me fulfill my commitment?

_____

_____

How can I hold myself accountable to this plan and track my progress?

_____

_____

Emotion List

Below is a list of feeling words, organized by category, to help you accurately label emotions in your daily journal reflections.

ANGER
- Annoyed
- Agitated
- Impatient
- Irritated
- Frustrated
- Resentful
- Furious
- Livid
- Enraged

SADNESS
- Disappointed
- Hurt
- Lonely
- Hopeless
- Helpless
- Despairing
- Miserable
- Grief
- Depressed

PLEASANT EMOTIONS
- Content
- Calm
- Relieved
- Joyful
- Hopeful
- Excited
- Proud
- Grateful
- Amazed

FEAR AND ANXIETY
- Uncertain
- Uneasy
- Nervous
- Doubtful
- Worried
- Apprehensive
- Panicked
- Afraid
- Terrified

GUILT AND SHAME
- Awkward
- Embarrassed
- Self-Conscious
- Regretful
- Vulnerable
- Offended
- Rejected
- Inferior
- Humiliated

MISC EMOTIONS
- Bored
- Numb
- Apathetic
- Confused
- Shocked
- Surprised
- Envious
- Jealous
- Disgusted

You'll also find an extended list of emotions at http://www.newharbinger.com/51963.

The Daily Journal

MINDFULNESS

START-OF-DAY REFLECTION   DATE

What emotions am I feeling and why?

_____

_____

_____

_____

_____

What's my goal today?

_____

_____

_____

_____

What might challenge me today? How can I be skillful?

_____

_____

_____

_____

_____

END-OF-DAY REFLECTION

How can I be less judgmental of my shortcomings and imperfections? What can I tell myself instead?

_____

_____

_____

_____

_____

_____

What did I accomplish or learn today? What am I grateful for?

_____

_____

_____

_____

_____

DBT SKILLS PRACTICED TODAY

MINDFULNESS	DISTRESS TOLERANCE	EMOTION REGULATION	INTERPERSONAL EFFECTIVENESS
_____	_____	_____	_____
_____	_____	_____	_____
_____	_____	_____	_____

START-OF-DAY REFLECTION

What emotions am I feeling and why?

_____

_____

_____

_____

_____

What's my goal today?

_____

_____

_____

_____

What might challenge me today? How can I be skillful?

_____

_____

_____

_____

_____

END-OF-DAY REFLECTION

How do I normally respond to strong, unpleasant emotions? Do I ever invalidate or blame myself for them? Where do these words or messages come from?

_____

_____

_____

_____

_____

_____

What did I accomplish or learn today? What am I grateful for?

_____

_____

_____

_____

_____

DBT SKILLS PRACTICED TODAY

MINDFULNESS	DISTRESS TOLERANCE	EMOTION REGULATION	INTERPERSONAL EFFECTIVENESS
_____	_____	_____	_____
_____	_____	_____	_____
_____	_____	_____	_____

START-OF-DAY REFLECTION DATE

What emotions am I feeling and why?

_____

_____

_____

_____

_____

What's my goal today?

_____

_____

_____

_____

What might challenge me today? How can I be skillful?

_____

_____

_____

_____

_____

END-OF-DAY REFLECTION

What was the last conflict or stressful situation I faced? What negative thoughts or judgments arose? What can I do with these thoughts next time they arise?

_____

_____

_____

_____

_____

_____

What did I accomplish or learn today? What am I grateful for?

_____

_____

_____

_____

DBT SKILLS PRACTICED TODAY

MINDFULNESS	DISTRESS TOLERANCE	EMOTION REGULATION	INTERPERSONAL EFFECTIVENESS
_____	_____	_____	_____
_____	_____	_____	_____
_____	_____	_____	_____

START-OF-DAY REFLECTION DATE

What emotions am I feeling and why?

_____

_____

_____

_____

_____

What's my goal today?

_____

_____

_____

_____

What might challenge me today? How can I be skillful?

_____

_____

_____

_____

_____

END-OF-DAY REFLECTION

Where can I consider including a momentary pause today or tomorrow to gain clarity, calmness, or control?

_____

_____

_____

_____

_____

_____

What did I accomplish or learn today? What am I grateful for?

_____

_____

_____

_____

_____

DBT SKILLS PRACTICED TODAY

MINDFULNESS	DISTRESS TOLERANCE	EMOTION REGULATION	INTERPERSONAL EFFECTIVENESS
_____	_____	_____	_____
_____	_____	_____	_____
_____	_____	_____	_____

START-OF-DAY REFLECTION DATE

What emotions am I feeling and why?

_____

_____

_____

_____

_____

What's my goal today?

_____

_____

_____

_____

What might challenge me today? How can I be skillful?

_____

_____

_____

_____

_____

_____

END-OF-DAY REFLECTION

Where does my mind typically go when it wanders? Into the past? The future?
How does this impact my emotions?

_____

_____

_____

_____

_____

_____

What did I accomplish or learn today? What am I grateful for?

_____

_____

_____

_____

_____

DBT SKILLS PRACTICED TODAY

MINDFULNESS	DISTRESS TOLERANCE	EMOTION REGULATION	INTERPERSONAL EFFECTIVENESS
_____	_____	_____	_____
_____	_____	_____	_____
_____	_____	_____	_____

START-OF-DAY REFLECTION DATE

What emotions am I feeling and why?

What's my goal today?

What might challenge me today? How can I be skillful?

28

END-OF-DAY REFLECTION

What types of interactions or activities can I throw myself into fully, without worry or concern of being judged by others?

_____

_____

_____

_____

_____

_____

What did I accomplish or learn today? What am I grateful for?

_____

_____

_____

_____

_____

DBT SKILLS PRACTICED TODAY

MINDFULNESS	DISTRESS TOLERANCE	EMOTION REGULATION	INTERPERSONAL EFFECTIVENESS
_____	_____	_____	_____
_____	_____	_____	_____
_____	_____	_____	_____

START-OF-DAY REFLECTION

What emotions am I feeling and why?

_____

_____

_____

_____

_____

What's my goal today?

_____

_____

_____

_____

What might challenge me today? How can I be skillful?

_____

_____

_____

_____

_____

END-OF-DAY REFLECTION

What experiences or activities awaken my present-moment awareness? What allows me to really *be* in these moments?

_____

_____

_____

_____

_____

_____

What did I accomplish or learn today? What am I grateful for?

_____

_____

_____

_____

_____

DBT SKILLS PRACTICED TODAY

MINDFULNESS	DISTRESS TOLERANCE	EMOTION REGULATION	INTERPERSONAL EFFECTIVENESS

START-OF-DAY REFLECTION

What emotions am I feeling and why?

_____

_____

_____

_____

_____

What's my goal today?

_____

_____

_____

_____

What might challenge me today? How can I be skillful?

_____

_____

_____

_____

_____

END-OF-DAY REFLECTION

What are important goals or values to remind myself of when my emotions come with strong problematic urges?

_____

_____

_____

_____

_____

_____

What did I accomplish or learn today? What am I grateful for?

_____

_____

_____

_____

_____

DBT SKILLS PRACTICED TODAY

MINDFULNESS	DISTRESS TOLERANCE	EMOTION REGULATION	INTERPERSONAL EFFECTIVENESS
_____	_____	_____	_____
_____	_____	_____	_____
_____	_____	_____	_____

START-OF-DAY REFLECTION DATE

What emotions am I feeling and why?

_____

_____

_____

_____

_____

What's my goal today?

_____

_____

_____

_____

What might challenge me today? How can I be skillful?

_____

_____

_____

_____

_____

END-OF-DAY REFLECTION

What supportive messages do I tell others who are struggling? Does this differ from the way I talk to myself and how?

_____

_____

_____

_____

_____

_____

_____

What did I accomplish or learn today? What am I grateful for?

_____

_____

_____

_____

_____

DBT SKILLS PRACTICED TODAY

MINDFULNESS	DISTRESS TOLERANCE	EMOTION REGULATION	INTERPERSONAL EFFECTIVENESS
● _____	● _____	● _____	● _____
● _____	● _____	● _____	● _____
● _____	● _____	● _____	● _____

START-OF-DAY REFLECTION

What emotions am I feeling and why?

_____

_____

_____

_____

_____

What's my goal today?

_____

_____

_____

_____

What might challenge me today? How can I be skillful?

_____

_____

_____

_____

_____

END-OF-DAY REFLECTION

Thinking back to a recent difficulty I experienced: What did I think about it?
How did I feel? And—what might a wise, effective response to such a difficulty
look like?

_____

_____

_____

_____

_____

What did I accomplish or learn today? What am I grateful for?

_____

_____

_____

_____

_____

DBT SKILLS PRACTICED TODAY

MINDFULNESS	DISTRESS TOLERANCE	EMOTION REGULATION	INTERPERSONAL EFFECTIVENESS
_____	_____	_____	_____
_____	_____	_____	_____
_____	_____	_____	_____

START-OF-DAY REFLECTION DATE

What emotions am I feeling and why?

What's my goal today?

What might challenge me today? How can I be skillful?

END-OF-DAY REFLECTION

When do I feel most compelled to judge myself or others harshly? What brings me to a more accepting stance toward myself or others?

_____

_____

_____

_____

_____

_____

_____

What did I accomplish or learn today? What am I grateful for?

_____

_____

_____

_____

_____

DBT SKILLS PRACTICED TODAY

MINDFULNESS	DISTRESS TOLERANCE	EMOTION REGULATION	INTERPERSONAL EFFECTIVENESS
_____	_____	_____	_____
_____	_____	_____	_____
_____	_____	_____	_____

START-OF-DAY REFLECTION

What emotions am I feeling and why?

What's my goal today?

What might challenge me today? How can I be skillful?

END-OF-DAY REFLECTION

What's a past struggle or failure my mind frequently wanders to? Is it effective to let my mind wander here? What can I do next time this happens?

_____

_____

_____

_____

_____

_____

_____

What did I accomplish or learn today? What am I grateful for?

_____

_____

_____

_____

_____

DBT SKILLS PRACTICED TODAY

MINDFULNESS	DISTRESS TOLERANCE	EMOTION REGULATION	INTERPERSONAL EFFECTIVENESS
_____	_____	_____	_____
_____	_____	_____	_____
_____	_____	_____	_____

START-OF-DAY REFLECTION

What emotions am I feeling and why?

_____

_____

_____

_____

_____

What's my goal today?

_____

_____

_____

_____

What might challenge me today? How can I be skillful?

_____

_____

_____

_____

_____

END-OF-DAY REFLECTION

Where in my life do I lack present-moment focus? What distracts me from the present moment?

_____

_____

_____

_____

_____

_____

_____

What did I accomplish or learn today? What am I grateful for?

_____

_____

_____

_____

_____

_____

DBT SKILLS PRACTICED TODAY

MINDFULNESS	DISTRESS TOLERANCE	EMOTION REGULATION	INTERPERSONAL EFFECTIVENESS
_____	_____	_____	_____
_____	_____	_____	_____
_____	_____	_____	_____

START-OF-DAY REFLECTION

What emotions am I feeling and why?

What's my goal today?

What might challenge me today? How can I be skillful?

END-OF-DAY REFLECTION

How can I cultivate more kindness in my thoughts, words, and actions toward myself or others?

_____

_____

_____

_____

_____

_____

What did I accomplish or learn today? What am I grateful for?

_____

_____

_____

_____

_____

DBT SKILLS PRACTICED TODAY

MINDFULNESS	DISTRESS TOLERANCE	EMOTION REGULATION	INTERPERSONAL EFFECTIVENESS
_____	_____	_____	_____
_____	_____	_____	_____
_____	_____	_____	_____

START-OF-DAY REFLECTION DATE

What emotions am I feeling and why?

_____

_____

_____

_____

_____

What's my goal today?

_____

_____

_____

_____

What might challenge me today? How can I be skillful?

_____

_____

_____

_____

_____

END-OF-DAY REFLECTION

When do I use self-judgment as a motivator for self-improvement? What is unhelpful about this?

_____

_____

_____

_____

_____

_____

What did I accomplish or learn today? What am I grateful for?

_____

_____

_____

_____

_____

DBT SKILLS PRACTICED TODAY

MINDFULNESS	DISTRESS TOLERANCE	EMOTION REGULATION	INTERPERSONAL EFFECTIVENESS
• _____	• _____	• _____	• _____
• _____	• _____	• _____	• _____
• _____	• _____	• _____	• _____

START-OF-DAY REFLECTION DATE

What emotions am I feeling and why?

_____

_____

_____

_____

_____

What's my goal today?

_____

_____

_____

_____

What might challenge me today? How can I be skillful?

_____

_____

_____

_____

END-OF-DAY REFLECTION

Where do I allow myself to go with the flow of things, with spontaneity and openness?

_____

_____

_____

_____

_____

_____

What did I accomplish or learn today? What am I grateful for?

_____

_____

_____

_____

_____

DBT SKILLS PRACTICED TODAY

MINDFULNESS	DISTRESS TOLERANCE	EMOTION REGULATION	INTERPERSONAL EFFECTIVENESS
_____	_____	_____	_____
_____	_____	_____	_____
_____	_____	_____	_____

START-OF-DAY REFLECTION

 DATE

What emotions am I feeling and why?

What's my goal today?

What might challenge me today? How can I be skillful?

END-OF-DAY REFLECTION

Where do my emotions misguide me with their sense of urgency? When do my emotions take control of my actions? What triggers these emotional reactions?

_____

_____

_____

_____

_____

_____

_____

What did I accomplish or learn today? What am I grateful for?

_____

_____

_____

_____

_____

DBT SKILLS PRACTICED TODAY

MINDFULNESS	DISTRESS TOLERANCE	EMOTION REGULATION	INTERPERSONAL EFFECTIVENESS
_____	_____	_____	_____
_____	_____	_____	_____
_____	_____	_____	_____

START-OF-DAY REFLECTION

What emotions am I feeling and why?

_____

_____

_____

_____

_____

What's my goal today?

_____

_____

_____

_____

What might challenge me today? How can I be skillful?

_____

_____

_____

_____

_____

END-OF-DAY REFLECTION

What am I noticing in my mind and body right now? What is this linked to? Do I find myself welcoming these experiences or pushing them away?

_____

_____

_____

_____

_____

_____

_____

What did I accomplish or learn today? What am I grateful for?

_____

_____

_____

_____

_____

DBT SKILLS PRACTICED TODAY

MINDFULNESS	DISTRESS TOLERANCE	EMOTION REGULATION	INTERPERSONAL EFFECTIVENESS
● _____	● _____	● _____	● _____
● _____	● _____	● _____	● _____
● _____	● _____	● _____	● _____

The Daily Journal

DISTRESS TOLERANCE

START-OF-DAY REFLECTION

What emotions am I feeling and why?

What's my goal today?

What might challenge me today? How can I be skillful?

END-OF-DAY REFLECTION

What are the signs of an emotional crisis that are unique to me and my circumstances? What are the most common triggers to these situations?

_____

_____

_____

_____

_____

_____

What did I accomplish or learn today? What am I grateful for?

_____

_____

_____

_____

_____

DBT SKILLS PRACTICED TODAY

MINDFULNESS	DISTRESS TOLERANCE	EMOTION REGULATION	INTERPERSONAL EFFECTIVENESS
_____	_____	_____	_____
_____	_____	_____	_____
_____	_____	_____	_____

START-OF-DAY REFLECTION

What emotions am I feeling and why?

_____

_____

_____

_____

_____

What's my goal today?

_____

_____

_____

_____

What might challenge me today? How can I be skillful?

_____

_____

_____

_____

_____

END-OF-DAY REFLECTION

When I notice body tension, what generally helps to ease and soothe the discomfort?

_____

_____

_____

_____

_____

_____

_____

What did I accomplish or learn today? What am I grateful for?

_____

_____

_____

_____

_____

DBT SKILLS PRACTICED TODAY

MINDFULNESS	DISTRESS TOLERANCE	EMOTION REGULATION	INTERPERSONAL EFFECTIVENESS
⦾ _____	⦾ _____	⦾ _____	⦾ _____
⦾ _____	⦾ _____	⦾ _____	⦾ _____
⦾ _____	⦾ _____	⦾ _____	⦾ _____

START-OF-DAY REFLECTION DATE

What emotions am I feeling and why?

What's my goal today?

What might challenge me today? How can I be skillful?

END-OF-DAY REFLECTION

Do I ever use distraction as a way to avoid my problems? Does this lead to more problems or worsen them? What are more effective temporary distractions?

_____

_____

_____

_____

_____

_____

What did I accomplish or learn today? What am I grateful for?

_____

_____

_____

_____

_____

DBT SKILLS PRACTICED TODAY

MINDFULNESS	DISTRESS TOLERANCE	EMOTION REGULATION	INTERPERSONAL EFFECTIVENESS
_____	_____	_____	_____
_____	_____	_____	_____
_____	_____	_____	_____

START-OF-DAY REFLECTION DATE

What emotions am I feeling and why?

_____

_____

_____

_____

_____

What's my goal today?

_____

_____

_____

_____

What might challenge me today? How can I be skillful?

_____

_____

_____

_____

_____

END-OF-DAY REFLECTION

What challenges have I overcome before that I am proud of? How can I use this as motivation to push through hard times in the future?

_____

_____

_____

_____

_____

_____

What did I accomplish or learn today? What am I grateful for?

_____

_____

_____

_____

DBT SKILLS PRACTICED TODAY

MINDFULNESS	DISTRESS TOLERANCE	EMOTION REGULATION	INTERPERSONAL EFFECTIVENESS
○ _____	○ _____	○ _____	○ _____
○ _____	○ _____	○ _____	○ _____
○ _____	○ _____	○ _____	○ _____

START-OF-DAY REFLECTION DATE

What emotions am I feeling and why?

What's my goal today?

What might challenge me today? How can I be skillful?

END-OF-DAY REFLECTION

What are the obstacles to fully accepting undesirable life events? What helps me persevere and not give up when life does not seem to be going the way I want it to?

_____

_____

_____

_____

_____

_____

What did I accomplish or learn today? What am I grateful for?

_____

_____

_____

_____

DBT SKILLS PRACTICED TODAY

MINDFULNESS	DISTRESS TOLERANCE	EMOTION REGULATION	INTERPERSONAL EFFECTIVENESS
_____	_____	_____	_____
_____	_____	_____	_____
_____	_____	_____	_____

START-OF-DAY REFLECTION DATE

What emotions am I feeling and why?

What's my goal today?

What might challenge me today? How can I be skillful?

END-OF-DAY REFLECTION

What unhelpful or negative thoughts arise during moments of distress? What are more useful thoughts to tell myself in these moments?

_____

_____

_____

_____

_____

_____

_____

What did I accomplish or learn today? What am I grateful for?

_____

_____

_____

_____

_____

DBT SKILLS PRACTICED TODAY

MINDFULNESS	DISTRESS TOLERANCE	EMOTION REGULATION	INTERPERSONAL EFFECTIVENESS
○ _____	○ _____	○ _____	○ _____
○ _____	○ _____	○ _____	○ _____
○ _____	○ _____	○ _____	○ _____

START-OF-DAY REFLECTION

What emotions am I feeling and why?

_____

_____

_____

_____

What's my goal today?

_____

_____

_____

What might challenge me today? How can I be skillful?

_____

_____

_____

_____

END-OF-DAY REFLECTION

In what current or future situations would it be helpful to pause and mindfully reflect about my intentions before taking any further action?

_____

_____

_____

_____

_____

_____

What did I accomplish or learn today? What am I grateful for?

_____

_____

_____

_____

_____

DBT SKILLS PRACTICED TODAY

MINDFULNESS	DISTRESS TOLERANCE	EMOTION REGULATION	INTERPERSONAL EFFECTIVENESS
_____	_____	_____	_____
_____	_____	_____	_____
_____	_____	_____	_____

START-OF-DAY REFLECTION DATE

What emotions am I feeling and why?

_____

_____

_____

_____

_____

_____

What's my goal today?

_____

_____

_____

_____

_____

What might challenge me today? How can I be skillful?

_____

_____

_____

_____

_____

END-OF-DAY REFLECTION

What is a recent difficult event that I fully accepted for what it was, without resistance? What made this possible?

_____

_____

_____

_____

_____

_____

What did I accomplish or learn today? What am I grateful for?

_____

_____

_____

_____

_____

DBT SKILLS PRACTICED TODAY

MINDFULNESS	DISTRESS TOLERANCE	EMOTION REGULATION	INTERPERSONAL EFFECTIVENESS
_____	_____	_____	_____
_____	_____	_____	_____
_____	_____	_____	_____

START-OF-DAY REFLECTION DATE

What emotions am I feeling and why?

_____

_____

_____

_____

_____

What's my goal today?

_____

_____

_____

_____

What might challenge me today? How can I be skillful?

_____

_____

_____

_____

_____

END-OF-DAY REFLECTION

What is a very memorable pleasant moment and why? When and how can I use this memory and savor the feelings the next time I'm struggling with something?

_____

_____

_____

_____

_____

_____

What did I accomplish or learn today? What am I grateful for?

_____

_____

_____

_____

_____

DBT SKILLS PRACTICED TODAY

MINDFULNESS	DISTRESS TOLERANCE	EMOTION REGULATION	INTERPERSONAL EFFECTIVENESS
_____	_____	_____	_____
_____	_____	_____	_____
_____	_____	_____	_____

START-OF-DAY REFLECTION

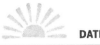

What emotions am I feeling and why?

What's my goal today?

What might challenge me today? How can I be skillful?

END-OF-DAY REFLECTION

What is my most positive vision for myself and my future? How can this vision guide me during challenging situations?

_____

_____

_____

_____

_____

_____

What did I accomplish or learn today? What am I grateful for?

_____

_____

_____

_____

_____

DBT SKILLS PRACTICED TODAY

MINDFULNESS	DISTRESS TOLERANCE	EMOTION REGULATION	INTERPERSONAL EFFECTIVENESS
_____	_____	_____	_____
_____	_____	_____	_____
_____	_____	_____	_____

START-OF-DAY REFLECTION DATE

What emotions am I feeling and why?

_____

_____

_____

_____

_____

What's my goal today?

_____

_____

_____

_____

What might challenge me today? How can I be skillful?

_____

_____

_____

_____

END-OF-DAY REFLECTION

What is my perfect combination of self-care routines to soothe myself?

_____

_____

_____

_____

_____

_____

_____

What did I accomplish or learn today? What am I grateful for?

_____

_____

_____

_____

_____

DBT SKILLS PRACTICED TODAY

MINDFULNESS	DISTRESS TOLERANCE	EMOTION REGULATION	INTERPERSONAL EFFECTIVENESS
_____	_____	_____	_____
_____	_____	_____	_____
_____	_____	_____	_____

START-OF-DAY REFLECTION DATE

What emotions am I feeling and why?

_____

_____

_____

_____

_____

What's my goal today?

_____

_____

_____

_____

What might challenge me today? How can I be skillful?

_____

_____

_____

_____

_____

END-OF-DAY REFLECTION

What are some situations where acting on my emotions feels good in the moment? What are both the positive and negative outcomes of doing so—short term and long term?

_____

_____

_____

_____

_____

_____

What did I accomplish or learn today? What am I grateful for?

_____

_____

_____

_____

_____

DBT SKILLS PRACTICED TODAY

MINDFULNESS	DISTRESS TOLERANCE	EMOTION REGULATION	INTERPERSONAL EFFECTIVENESS
_____	_____	_____	_____
_____	_____	_____	_____
_____	_____	_____	_____

START-OF-DAY REFLECTION

What emotions am I feeling and why?

_____

_____

_____

_____

_____

What's my goal today?

_____

_____

_____

_____

What might challenge me today? How can I be skillful?

_____

_____

_____

_____

END-OF-DAY REFLECTION

When does tolerating and accepting certain problems or difficulties work better than trying to fix, control, or change them?

_____

_____

_____

_____

_____

_____

What did I accomplish or learn today? What am I grateful for?

_____

_____

_____

_____

_____

DBT SKILLS PRACTICED TODAY

MINDFULNESS	DISTRESS TOLERANCE	EMOTION REGULATION	INTERPERSONAL EFFECTIVENESS
_____	_____	_____	_____
_____	_____	_____	_____
_____	_____	_____	_____

START-OF-DAY REFLECTION DATE

What emotions am I feeling and why?

_____

_____

_____

_____

_____

What's my goal today?

_____

_____

_____

_____

What might challenge me today? How can I be skillful?

_____

_____

_____

_____

_____

END-OF-DAY REFLECTION

What unhelpful behaviors do I engage in to escape painful emotions? What emotions do I avoid the most and why? What would be an alternative effective approach to these emotions?

_____

_____

_____

_____

_____

What did I accomplish or learn today? What am I grateful for?

_____

_____

_____

_____

_____

DBT SKILLS PRACTICED TODAY

MINDFULNESS	DISTRESS TOLERANCE	EMOTION REGULATION	INTERPERSONAL EFFECTIVENESS
_____	_____	_____	_____
_____	_____	_____	_____
_____	_____	_____	_____

START-OF-DAY REFLECTION

What emotions am I feeling and why?

_____

_____

_____

_____

_____

What's my goal today?

_____

_____

_____

_____

_____

What might challenge me today? How can I be skillful?

_____

_____

_____

_____

_____

_____

END-OF-DAY REFLECTION

What makes my life fulfilling and meaningful, even with painful or stressful circumstances in it?

_____

_____

_____

_____

_____

_____

_____

What did I accomplish or learn today? What am I grateful for?

_____

_____

_____

_____

_____

DBT SKILLS PRACTICED TODAY

MINDFULNESS	DISTRESS TOLERANCE	EMOTION REGULATION	INTERPERSONAL EFFECTIVENESS
_____	_____	_____	_____
_____	_____	_____	_____
_____	_____	_____	_____

START-OF-DAY REFLECTION

What emotions am I feeling and why?

What's my goal today?

What might challenge me today? How can I be skillful?

END-OF-DAY REFLECTION

When is it wiser to tolerate my emotional urges than to act on them? What goals can I set and what skills can I use to help me tolerate them? What are the benefits of doing so?

_____

_____

_____

_____

_____

_____

What did I accomplish or learn today? What am I grateful for?

_____

_____

_____

_____

_____

DBT SKILLS PRACTICED TODAY

MINDFULNESS	DISTRESS TOLERANCE	EMOTION REGULATION	INTERPERSONAL EFFECTIVENESS
_____	_____	_____	_____
_____	_____	_____	_____
_____	_____	_____	_____

START-OF-DAY REFLECTION

What emotions am I feeling and why?

_____

_____

_____

_____

_____

What's my goal today?

_____

_____

_____

_____

What might challenge me today? How can I be skillful?

_____

_____

_____

_____

_____

END-OF-DAY REFLECTION

What is happening or what has happened in my life that I have difficulty letting go of, and why? Which of these are out of my control? What can I let go of trying to control and how?

_____

_____

_____

_____

_____

_____

What did I accomplish or learn today? What am I grateful for?

_____

_____

_____

_____

_____

DBT SKILLS PRACTICED TODAY

MINDFULNESS	DISTRESS TOLERANCE	EMOTION REGULATION	INTERPERSONAL EFFECTIVENESS
● _____	● _____	● _____	● _____
● _____	● _____	● _____	● _____
● _____	● _____	● _____	● _____

START-OF-DAY REFLECTION

What emotions am I feeling and why?

_____

_____

_____

_____

_____

_____

What's my goal today?

_____

_____

_____

_____

_____

What might challenge me today? How can I be skillful?

_____

_____

_____

_____

_____

_____

END-OF-DAY REFLECTION

What encouraging phrases or positive affirmations do I need to hear from myself or others to help me get through difficult or distressing moments?

_____

_____

_____

_____

_____

_____

What did I accomplish or learn today? What am I grateful for?

_____

_____

_____

_____

_____

DBT SKILLS PRACTICED TODAY

MINDFULNESS	DISTRESS TOLERANCE	EMOTION REGULATION	INTERPERSONAL EFFECTIVENESS
_____	_____	_____	_____
_____	_____	_____	_____
_____	_____	_____	_____

The Daily Journal

EMOTION REGULATION

START-OF-DAY REFLECTION

What emotions am I feeling and why?

What's my goal today?

What might challenge me today? How can I be skillful?

END-OF-DAY REFLECTION

What situations regularly bring up anger or frustration? Does the intensity of these emotions seem to match the situations in the moment? Why or why not?

What did I accomplish or learn today? What am I grateful for?

DBT SKILLS PRACTICED TODAY

MINDFULNESS	DISTRESS TOLERANCE	EMOTION REGULATION	INTERPERSONAL EFFECTIVENESS

START-OF-DAY REFLECTION 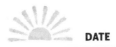 DATE

What emotions am I feeling and why?

What's my goal today?

What might challenge me today? How can I be skillful?

END-OF-DAY REFLECTION

What is one short- or long-term problem that needs to be solved soon? What is my goal and what potential solutions are there to solve this?

_____

_____

_____

_____

_____

_____

What did I accomplish or learn today? What am I grateful for?

_____

_____

_____

_____

_____

DBT SKILLS PRACTICED TODAY

MINDFULNESS	DISTRESS TOLERANCE	EMOTION REGULATION	INTERPERSONAL EFFECTIVENESS
_____	_____	_____	_____
_____	_____	_____	_____
_____	_____	_____	_____

START-OF-DAY REFLECTION 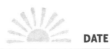 DATE

What emotions am I feeling and why?

What's my goal today?

What might challenge me today? How can I be skillful?

98

END-OF-DAY REFLECTION

Where do my judgments interfere with seeing things as they really are? Do my emotions ever influence more rigid and inaccurate judgments?

_____

_____

_____

_____

_____

_____

What did I accomplish or learn today? What am I grateful for?

_____

_____

_____

_____

_____

DBT SKILLS PRACTICED TODAY

MINDFULNESS	DISTRESS TOLERANCE	EMOTION REGULATION	INTERPERSONAL EFFECTIVENESS
_____	_____	_____	_____
_____	_____	_____	_____
_____	_____	_____	_____

START-OF-DAY REFLECTION

What emotions am I feeling and why?

What's my goal today?

What might challenge me today? How can I be skillful?

END-OF-DAY REFLECTION

In what ways do my emotions help me—short term and long term? In what ways do they hinder my well-being?

_____

_____

_____

_____

_____

_____

What did I accomplish or learn today? What am I grateful for?

_____

_____

_____

_____

_____

DBT SKILLS PRACTICED TODAY

MINDFULNESS	DISTRESS TOLERANCE	EMOTION REGULATION	INTERPERSONAL EFFECTIVENESS
_____	_____	_____	_____
_____	_____	_____	_____
_____	_____	_____	_____

START-OF-DAY REFLECTION DATE

What emotions am I feeling and why?

_____

_____

_____

_____

_____

What's my goal today?

_____

_____

_____

_____

What might challenge me today? How can I be skillful?

_____

_____

_____

_____

_____

END-OF-DAY REFLECTION

If I did not fear failure, what would I be doing differently in my life? What can I do to act opposite to this fear?

_____

_____

_____

_____

_____

_____

What did I accomplish or learn today? What am I grateful for?

_____

_____

_____

_____

_____

DBT SKILLS PRACTICED TODAY

MINDFULNESS	DISTRESS TOLERANCE	EMOTION REGULATION	INTERPERSONAL EFFECTIVENESS
○ _____	○ _____	○ _____	○ _____
○ _____	○ _____	○ _____	○ _____
○ _____	○ _____	○ _____	○ _____

START-OF-DAY REFLECTION DATE

What emotions am I feeling and why?

What's my goal today?

What might challenge me today? How can I be skillful?

END-OF-DAY REFLECTION

In what ways does taking care of my physical health improve my mental and emotional health? What physical health needs do I neglect and what do I need to do more of?

_____

_____

_____

_____

_____

What did I accomplish or learn today? What am I grateful for?

_____

_____

_____

_____

_____

DBT SKILLS PRACTICED TODAY

MINDFULNESS	DISTRESS TOLERANCE	EMOTION REGULATION	INTERPERSONAL EFFECTIVENESS
● _____	● _____	● _____	● _____
● _____	● _____	● _____	● _____
● _____	● _____	● _____	● _____

START-OF-DAY REFLECTION DATE

What emotions am I feeling and why?

_____

_____

_____

_____

_____

What's my goal today?

_____

_____

_____

_____

What might challenge me today? How can I be skillful?

_____

_____

_____

_____

_____

END-OF-DAY REFLECTION

What do I find most difficult about attending to difficult emotions? What coping strategies typically support me in making space for these emotions?

_____

_____

_____

_____

_____

_____

What did I accomplish or learn today? What am I grateful for?

_____

_____

_____

_____

_____

DBT SKILLS PRACTICED TODAY

MINDFULNESS	DISTRESS TOLERANCE	EMOTION REGULATION	INTERPERSONAL EFFECTIVENESS
_____	_____	_____	_____
_____	_____	_____	_____
_____	_____	_____	_____

START-OF-DAY REFLECTION DATE

What emotions am I feeling and why?

_____

_____

_____

_____

_____

What's my goal today?

_____

_____

_____

_____

What might challenge me today? How can I be skillful?

_____

_____

_____

_____

_____

_____

END-OF-DAY REFLECTION

What is one pleasant experience that happened this week (minor or major) that made me smile? Where might there be more opportunities to cherish joyful or pleasurable moments like these?

_____

_____

_____

_____

_____

_____

What did I accomplish or learn today? What am I grateful for?

_____

_____

_____

_____

_____

DBT SKILLS PRACTICED TODAY

MINDFULNESS	DISTRESS TOLERANCE	EMOTION REGULATION	INTERPERSONAL EFFECTIVENESS
_____	_____	_____	_____
_____	_____	_____	_____
_____	_____	_____	_____

START-OF-DAY REFLECTION DATE

What emotions am I feeling and why?

_____

_____

_____

_____

_____

_____

What's my goal today?

_____

_____

_____

_____

What might challenge me today? How can I be skillful?

_____

_____

_____

_____

_____

END-OF-DAY REFLECTION

What coping strategies help me most when I feel too upset to use coping skills and want to default to ineffective ways of coping?

_____

_____

_____

_____

_____

_____

What did I accomplish or learn today? What am I grateful for?

_____

_____

_____

_____

_____

DBT SKILLS PRACTICED TODAY

MINDFULNESS	DISTRESS TOLERANCE	EMOTION REGULATION	INTERPERSONAL EFFECTIVENESS
_____	_____	_____	_____
_____	_____	_____	_____
_____	_____	_____	_____

START-OF-DAY REFLECTION

DATE

What emotions am I feeling and why?

What's my goal today?

What might challenge me today? How can I be skillful?

END-OF-DAY REFLECTION

What emotions do I try to avoid, not feel, or hide from others and why? How would I ideally wish to experience my emotions and how can I do this instead?

_____

_____

_____

_____

_____

_____

_____

What did I accomplish or learn today? What am I grateful for?

_____

_____

_____

_____

_____

DBT SKILLS PRACTICED TODAY

MINDFULNESS	DISTRESS TOLERANCE	EMOTION REGULATION	INTERPERSONAL EFFECTIVENESS
_____	_____	_____	_____
_____	_____	_____	_____
_____	_____	_____	_____

START-OF-DAY REFLECTION DATE

What emotions am I feeling and why?

_____

_____

_____

_____

_____

What's my goal today?

_____

_____

_____

_____

What might challenge me today? How can I be skillful?

_____

_____

_____

_____

_____

END-OF-DAY REFLECTION

What is an important value of mine that brings me gratification and fulfillment? How am I currently fulfilling this value, or not?

_____

_____

_____

_____

_____

_____

What did I accomplish or learn today? What am I grateful for?

_____

_____

_____

_____

_____

DBT SKILLS PRACTICED TODAY

MINDFULNESS	DISTRESS TOLERANCE	EMOTION REGULATION	INTERPERSONAL EFFECTIVENESS
_____	_____	_____	_____
_____	_____	_____	_____
_____	_____	_____	_____

START-OF-DAY REFLECTION

What emotions am I feeling and why?

What's my goal today?

What might challenge me today? How can I be skillful?

END-OF-DAY REFLECTION

What is a worst-case-scenario worry that I often think about? What are the ways I would cope with or solve it if it were to actually happen, no matter how stressful it might be?

_____

_____

_____

_____

_____

_____

What did I accomplish or learn today? What am I grateful for?

_____

_____

_____

_____

_____

DBT SKILLS PRACTICED TODAY

MINDFULNESS	DISTRESS TOLERANCE	EMOTION REGULATION	INTERPERSONAL EFFECTIVENESS
_____	_____	_____	_____
_____	_____	_____	_____
_____	_____	_____	_____

START-OF-DAY REFLECTION DATE

What emotions am I feeling and why?

_____

_____

_____

_____

_____

What's my goal today?

_____

_____

_____

_____

What might challenge me today? How can I be skillful?

_____

_____

_____

_____

_____

END-OF-DAY REFLECTION

What is an upcoming challenge I have to face? What coping skills can I plan to use to help me get through this?

_____

_____

_____

_____

_____

_____

_____

What did I accomplish or learn today? What am I grateful for?

_____

_____

_____

_____

_____

DBT SKILLS PRACTICED TODAY

MINDFULNESS	DISTRESS TOLERANCE	EMOTION REGULATION	INTERPERSONAL EFFECTIVENESS
_____	_____	_____	_____
_____	_____	_____	_____
_____	_____	_____	_____

START-OF-DAY REFLECTION

What emotions am I feeling and why?

_____

_____

_____

_____

_____

What's my goal today?

_____

_____

_____

_____

What might challenge me today? How can I be skillful?

_____

_____

_____

_____

_____

END-OF-DAY REFLECTION

What is a worry I frequently have? What are all possible outcomes for this situation? How likely is it that the worry will *really* come true?

_____

_____

_____

_____

_____

_____

_____

What did I accomplish or learn today? What am I grateful for?

_____

_____

_____

_____

_____

DBT SKILLS PRACTICED TODAY

MINDFULNESS	DISTRESS TOLERANCE	EMOTION REGULATION	INTERPERSONAL EFFECTIVENESS
○ _____	○ _____	○ _____	○ _____
○ _____	○ _____	○ _____	○ _____
○ _____	○ _____	○ _____	○ _____

START-OF-DAY REFLECTION DATE

What emotions am I feeling and why?

_____

_____

_____

_____

_____

What's my goal today?

_____

_____

_____

_____

What might challenge me today? How can I be skillful?

_____

_____

_____

_____

_____

END-OF-DAY REFLECTION

What are my views on expressing emotions to others? Does this change
when it's my emotions versus someone else's? How does this impact my own
emotional expression?

_____

_____

_____

_____

_____

_____

What did I accomplish or learn today? What am I grateful for?

_____

_____

_____

_____

_____

DBT SKILLS PRACTICED TODAY

MINDFULNESS	DISTRESS TOLERANCE	EMOTION REGULATION	INTERPERSONAL EFFECTIVENESS
● _____	● _____	● _____	● _____
● _____	● _____	● _____	● _____
● _____	● _____	● _____	● _____

START-OF-DAY REFLECTION

What emotions am I feeling and why?

_____

_____

_____

_____

_____

_____

What's my goal today?

_____

_____

_____

_____

_____

What might challenge me today? How can I be skillful?

_____

_____

_____

_____

_____

END-OF-DAY REFLECTION

What is something about myself that I hide from others, that others might actually accept me for? Who in my life would accept me for this?

_____

_____

_____

_____

_____

_____

What did I accomplish or learn today? What am I grateful for?

_____

_____

_____

_____

_____

DBT SKILLS PRACTICED TODAY

MINDFULNESS	DISTRESS TOLERANCE	EMOTION REGULATION	INTERPERSONAL EFFECTIVENESS

START-OF-DAY REFLECTION

DATE

What emotions am I feeling and why?

_____

_____

_____

_____

_____

What's my goal today?

_____

_____

_____

_____

_____

What might challenge me today? How can I be skillful?

_____

_____

_____

_____

_____

END-OF-DAY REFLECTION

What activities make me feel most accomplished and proud of myself? Where in my routine can I integrate more activities that give me these feelings?

_____

_____

_____

_____

_____

_____

What did I accomplish or learn today? What am I grateful for?

_____

_____

_____

_____

_____

DBT SKILLS PRACTICED TODAY

MINDFULNESS	DISTRESS TOLERANCE	EMOTION REGULATION	INTERPERSONAL EFFECTIVENESS
○ _____	○ _____	○ _____	○ _____
○ _____	○ _____	○ _____	○ _____
○ _____	○ _____	○ _____	○ _____

START-OF-DAY REFLECTION

What emotions am I feeling and why?

What's my goal today?

What might challenge me today? How can I be skillful?

END-OF-DAY REFLECTION

What does my fear or worry get in the way of? What am I avoiding because of this? What can I do with this insight?

_____

_____

_____

_____

_____

_____

_____

What did I accomplish or learn today? What am I grateful for?

_____

_____

_____

_____

_____

_____

DBT SKILLS PRACTICED TODAY

MINDFULNESS	DISTRESS TOLERANCE	EMOTION REGULATION	INTERPERSONAL EFFECTIVENESS
_____	_____	_____	_____
_____	_____	_____	_____
_____	_____	_____	_____

The Daily Journal

INTERPERSONAL EFFECTIVENESS

START-OF-DAY REFLECTION DATE

What emotions am I feeling and why?

What's my goal today?

What might challenge me today? How can I be skillful?

END-OF-DAY REFLECTION

Who is someone I really admire? What does this say about the strengths, qualities, or values that are most important to me?

_____

_____

_____

_____

_____

_____

_____

What did I accomplish or learn today? What am I grateful for?

_____

_____

_____

_____

_____

_____

DBT SKILLS PRACTICED TODAY

MINDFULNESS	DISTRESS TOLERANCE	EMOTION REGULATION	INTERPERSONAL EFFECTIVENESS
○ _____	○ _____	○ _____	○ _____
○ _____	○ _____	○ _____	○ _____
○ _____	○ _____	○ _____	○ _____

START-OF-DAY REFLECTION

DATE

What emotions am I feeling and why?

_____

_____

_____

_____

_____

_____

What's my goal today?

_____

_____

_____

_____

_____

What might challenge me today? How can I be skillful?

_____

_____

_____

_____

_____

_____

END-OF-DAY REFLECTION

How do I handle expected and unexpected changes? What helps me embrace change, without resistance?

_____

_____

_____

_____

_____

_____

What did I accomplish or learn today? What am I grateful for?

_____

_____

_____

_____

_____

DBT SKILLS PRACTICED TODAY

MINDFULNESS	DISTRESS TOLERANCE	EMOTION REGULATION	INTERPERSONAL EFFECTIVENESS
● _____	● _____	● _____	● _____
● _____	● _____	● _____	● _____
● _____	● _____	● _____	● _____

START-OF-DAY REFLECTION DATE

What emotions am I feeling and why?

_____

_____

_____

_____

_____

What's my goal today?

_____

_____

_____

_____

What might challenge me today? How can I be skillful?

_____

_____

_____

_____

_____

END-OF-DAY REFLECTION

What do I need in my current relationships in order for me to be happy? What actions or changes, if any, are needed to make this happen?

_____

_____

_____

_____

_____

_____

What did I accomplish or learn today? What am I grateful for?

_____

_____

_____

_____

_____

DBT SKILLS PRACTICED TODAY

MINDFULNESS	DISTRESS TOLERANCE	EMOTION REGULATION	INTERPERSONAL EFFECTIVENESS
_____	_____	_____	_____
_____	_____	_____	_____
_____	_____	_____	_____

START-OF-DAY REFLECTION DATE

What emotions am I feeling and why?

_____

_____

_____

_____

_____

What's my goal today?

_____

_____

_____

_____

What might challenge me today? How can I be skillful?

_____

_____

_____

_____

_____

END-OF-DAY REFLECTION

When have I spoken up for myself and felt confident or proud? What made this possible?

_____

_____

_____

_____

_____

_____

What did I accomplish or learn today? What am I grateful for?

_____

_____

_____

_____

_____

DBT SKILLS PRACTICED TODAY

MINDFULNESS	DISTRESS TOLERANCE	EMOTION REGULATION	INTERPERSONAL EFFECTIVENESS
_____	_____	_____	_____
_____	_____	_____	_____
_____	_____	_____	_____

START-OF-DAY REFLECTION

What emotions am I feeling and why?

What's my goal today?

What might challenge me today? How can I be skillful?

END-OF-DAY REFLECTION

What makes me feel most deeply connected to others, even when they're not present? What, if anything, gets in the way?

_____

_____

_____

_____

_____

_____

What did I accomplish or learn today? What am I grateful for?

_____

_____

_____

_____

_____

DBT SKILLS PRACTICED TODAY

MINDFULNESS	DISTRESS TOLERANCE	EMOTION REGULATION	INTERPERSONAL EFFECTIVENESS
_____	_____	_____	_____
_____	_____	_____	_____
_____	_____	_____	_____

START-OF-DAY REFLECTION   DATE

What emotions am I feeling and why?

What's my goal today?

What might challenge me today? How can I be skillful?

END-OF-DAY REFLECTION

How do I handle conflict or confrontation with others? What helps me address and resolve these situations effectively?

_____

_____

_____

_____

_____

_____

What did I accomplish or learn today? What am I grateful for?

_____

_____

_____

_____

_____

DBT SKILLS PRACTICED TODAY

MINDFULNESS	DISTRESS TOLERANCE	EMOTION REGULATION	INTERPERSONAL EFFECTIVENESS
● _____	● _____	● _____	● _____
● _____	● _____	● _____	● _____
● _____	● _____	● _____	● _____

START-OF-DAY REFLECTION

What emotions am I feeling and why?

_____

_____

_____

_____

_____

What's my goal today?

_____

_____

_____

_____

What might challenge me today? How can I be skillful?

_____

_____

_____

_____

_____

END-OF-DAY REFLECTION

What is something I regret saying in the past? What would I change about what I said and how I said it?

_____

_____

_____

_____

_____

_____

What did I accomplish or learn today? What am I grateful for?

_____

_____

_____

_____

_____

DBT SKILLS PRACTICED TODAY

MINDFULNESS	DISTRESS TOLERANCE	EMOTION REGULATION	INTERPERSONAL EFFECTIVENESS
● _____	● _____	● _____	● _____
● _____	● _____	● _____	● _____
● _____	● _____	● _____	● _____

START-OF-DAY REFLECTION

DATE

What emotions am I feeling and why?

_____

_____

_____

_____

_____

What's my goal today?

_____

_____

_____

_____

What might challenge me today? How can I be skillful?

_____

_____

_____

_____

_____

Thinking back to a past disagreement or conflict involving another person: Can I factually describe this, without judgment? What is understandable about both their point of view and mine?

_____

_____

_____

_____

_____

_____

What did I accomplish or learn today? What am I grateful for?

_____

_____

_____

_____

_____

DBT SKILLS PRACTICED TODAY

MINDFULNESS	DISTRESS TOLERANCE	EMOTION REGULATION	INTERPERSONAL EFFECTIVENESS

START-OF-DAY REFLECTION

DATE

What emotions am I feeling and why?

What's my goal today?

What might challenge me today? How can I be skillful?

END-OF-DAY REFLECTION

How do I want others to view me? How would they view me today? What needs
to happen so that I am acting consistently with how I want to be viewed?

_____

_____

_____

_____

_____

_____

What did I accomplish or learn today? What am I grateful for?

_____

_____

_____

_____

_____

DBT SKILLS PRACTICED TODAY

MINDFULNESS	DISTRESS TOLERANCE	EMOTION REGULATION	INTERPERSONAL EFFECTIVENESS
○ _____	○ _____	○ _____	○ _____
○ _____	○ _____	○ _____	○ _____
○ _____	○ _____	○ _____	○ _____

149

START-OF-DAY REFLECTION DATE

What emotions am I feeling and why?

_____

_____

_____

_____

_____

What's my goal today?

_____

_____

_____

_____

What might challenge me today? How can I be skillful?

_____

_____

_____

_____

_____

_____

END-OF-DAY REFLECTION

Do I give others my full, undivided attention? What interferes with my full presence when around others?

_____

_____

_____

_____

_____

_____

What did I accomplish or learn today? What am I grateful for?

_____

_____

_____

_____

_____

DBT SKILLS PRACTICED TODAY

MINDFULNESS	DISTRESS TOLERANCE	EMOTION REGULATION	INTERPERSONAL EFFECTIVENESS
_____	_____	_____	_____
_____	_____	_____	_____
_____	_____	_____	_____

START-OF-DAY REFLECTION

What emotions am I feeling and why?

What's my goal today?

What might challenge me today? How can I be skillful?

END-OF-DAY REFLECTION

Where do I give more than what I get out of my relationships and at what expense? In what relationships is there a healthy balance?

_____

_____

_____

_____

_____

_____

What did I accomplish or learn today? What am I grateful for?

_____

_____

_____

_____

_____

DBT SKILLS PRACTICED TODAY

MINDFULNESS	DISTRESS TOLERANCE	EMOTION REGULATION	INTERPERSONAL EFFECTIVENESS
_____	_____	_____	_____
_____	_____	_____	_____
_____	_____	_____	_____

START-OF-DAY REFLECTION DATE

What emotions am I feeling and why?

_____

_____

_____

_____

_____

What's my goal today?

_____

_____

_____

_____

What might challenge me today? How can I be skillful?

_____

_____

_____

_____

_____

END-OF-DAY REFLECTION

What have I learned from previous relationship struggles or endings? How can this inform my present or future relationships?

_____

_____

_____

_____

_____

_____

_____

What did I accomplish or learn today? What am I grateful for?

_____

_____

_____

_____

_____

DBT SKILLS PRACTICED TODAY

MINDFULNESS	DISTRESS TOLERANCE	EMOTION REGULATION	INTERPERSONAL EFFECTIVENESS
_____	_____	_____	_____
_____	_____	_____	_____
_____	_____	_____	_____

START-OF-DAY REFLECTION DATE

What emotions am I feeling and why?

_____

_____

_____

_____

_____

What's my goal today?

_____

_____

_____

_____

What might challenge me today? How can I be skillful?

_____

_____

_____

_____

_____

END-OF-DAY REFLECTION

How do I make a positive impact in the lives of others? How can I continue to do more of this?

_____

_____

_____

_____

_____

_____

What did I accomplish or learn today? What am I grateful for?

_____

_____

_____

_____

_____

DBT SKILLS PRACTICED TODAY

MINDFULNESS	DISTRESS TOLERANCE	EMOTION REGULATION	INTERPERSONAL EFFECTIVENESS
● _____	● _____	● _____	● _____
● _____	● _____	● _____	● _____
● _____	● _____	● _____	● _____

START-OF-DAY REFLECTION

What emotions am I feeling and why?

_____

_____

_____

_____

_____

What's my goal today?

_____

_____

_____

_____

What might challenge me today? How can I be skillful?

_____

_____

_____

_____

_____

END-OF-DAY REFLECTION

What are the words I needed to hear most growing up? What can I say to myself to offer myself this same guidance from within?

_____

_____

_____

_____

_____

_____

What did I accomplish or learn today? What am I grateful for?

_____

_____

_____

_____

_____

DBT SKILLS PRACTICED TODAY

MINDFULNESS	DISTRESS TOLERANCE	EMOTION REGULATION	INTERPERSONAL EFFECTIVENESS
○ _____	○ _____	○ _____	○ _____
○ _____	○ _____	○ _____	○ _____
○ _____	○ _____	○ _____	○ _____

START-OF-DAY REFLECTION

What emotions am I feeling and why?

What's my goal today?

What might challenge me today? How can I be skillful?

END-OF-DAY REFLECTION

Looking around, what in the environment that I'm currently in signifies my connection to other beings?

_____

_____

_____

_____

_____

_____

What did I accomplish or learn today? What am I grateful for?

_____

_____

_____

_____

_____

DBT SKILLS PRACTICED TODAY

MINDFULNESS	DISTRESS TOLERANCE	EMOTION REGULATION	INTERPERSONAL EFFECTIVENESS

START-OF-DAY REFLECTION

What emotions am I feeling and why?

What's my goal today?

What might challenge me today? How can I be skillful?

END-OF-DAY REFLECTION

What are my tendencies when asking others for what I need or want? What are my tendencies when saying no to others? What can I do with these insights?

_____

_____

_____

_____

_____

_____

_____

What did I accomplish or learn today? What am I grateful for?

_____

_____

_____

_____

_____

_____

DBT SKILLS PRACTICED TODAY

MINDFULNESS	DISTRESS TOLERANCE	EMOTION REGULATION	INTERPERSONAL EFFECTIVENESS
● _____	● _____	● _____	● _____
● _____	● _____	● _____	● _____
● _____	● _____	● _____	● _____

START-OF-DAY REFLECTION

What emotions am I feeling and why?

_____

_____

_____

_____

_____

What's my goal today?

_____

_____

_____

_____

What might challenge me today? How can I be skillful?

_____

_____

_____

_____

_____

_____

END-OF-DAY REFLECTION

Who in my life is most accepting of me and allows me to be most vulnerable when I'm feeling guilty, ashamed, or withdrawn from others?

_____

_____

_____

_____

_____

_____

_____

What did I accomplish or learn today? What am I grateful for?

_____

_____

_____

_____

_____

DBT SKILLS PRACTICED TODAY

MINDFULNESS	DISTRESS TOLERANCE	EMOTION REGULATION	INTERPERSONAL EFFECTIVENESS
● _____	● _____	● _____	● _____
● _____	● _____	● _____	● _____
● _____	● _____	● _____	● _____

START-OF-DAY REFLECTION DATE

What emotions am I feeling and why?

_____

_____

_____

_____

_____

What's my goal today?

_____

_____

_____

_____

What might challenge me today? How can I be skillful?

_____

_____

_____

_____

_____

END-OF-DAY REFLECTION

What are the words or validation I have been longing to hear from someone influential in my life? Why is this important to me?

_____

_____

_____

_____

_____

_____

What did I accomplish or learn today? What am I grateful for?

_____

_____

_____

_____

DBT SKILLS PRACTICED TODAY

MINDFULNESS	DISTRESS TOLERANCE	EMOTION REGULATION	INTERPERSONAL EFFECTIVENESS
● _____	● _____	● _____	● _____
● _____	● _____	● _____	● _____
● _____	● _____	● _____	● _____

References

Emmons, B., and M.E. McCullough. 2003. "Counting Blessings Versus Burdens: An Experimental Investigation of Gratitude and Subjective Well-being in Daily Life." *Journal of Personality and Social Psychology* 84(2): 377–89.

Linehan, M. 1993. *Cognitive Behavioral Therapy for Borderline Personality Disorder*. New York: Guilford Press.

Linehan, M. 2014. *DBT Skills Training Manual*, 2nd ed. New York: Guilford Press.

Seligman, M. E., T. A. Steen, N. Park, and C. Peterson. 2005. "Positive Psychology Progress: Empirical Validation of Interventions." *American Psychologist* 60(5): 410–21.

Smyth, J. M., J. A. Johnson, B. J. Auer, E. Lehman, G. Talamo, and C. N. Sciamanna. 2018. "Online Positive Affect Journaling in the Improvement of Mental Distress and Well-being in General Medical Patients with Elevated Anxiety Symptoms: A Preliminary Randomized Controlled Trial." *JMIR Mental Health* 5(4): e11290.

DYLAN ZAMBRANO, MSW, is founder and clinical director of DBT Virtual, an online dialectical behavior therapy (DBT) service based in Ontario, Canada. He has several years of experience working on a DBT team within an outpatient mental health hospital setting, and provides DBT training, consultation, and supervision to other therapists. Dylan also teaches university continuing education courses and workshops in mindfulness and compassion meditation for health care professionals.

Foreword writer **SHERI VAN DIJK, MSW**, is a psychotherapist, renowned DBT expert, and author of several books, including *Don't Let Your Emotions Run Your Life for Teens*. Her books focus on using DBT skills to help people manage their emotions and cultivate lasting well-being.

MORE BOOKS from
NEW HARBINGER PUBLICATIONS

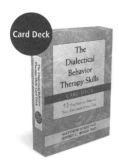

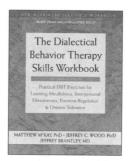

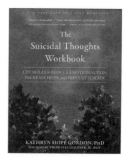

THE DIALECTICAL BEHAVIOR THERAPY CARD DECK

52 Practices to Balance Your Emotions Every Day

978-1684033980 / US $18.95

THE DIALECTICAL BEHAVIOR THERAPY SKILLS WORKBOOK, SECOND EDITION

Practical DBT Exercises for Learning Mindfulness, Interpersonal Effectiveness, Emotion Regulation, and Distress Tolerance

978-1684034581 / US $24.95

THE SUICIDAL THOUGHTS WORKBOOK

CBT Skills to Reduce Emotional Pain, Increase Hope, and Prevent Suicide

978-1684037025 / US $21.95

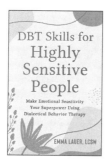

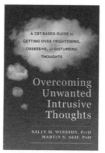

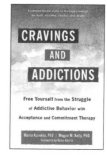

DBT SKILLS FOR HIGHLY SENSITIVE PEOPLE

Make Emotional Sensitivity Your Superpower Using Dialectical Behavior Therapy

978-1648481055 / US $18.95

OVERCOMING UNWANTED INTRUSIVE THOUGHTS

A CBT-Based Guide to Getting Over Frightening, Obsessive, or Disturbing Thoughts

978-1626254343 / US $17.95

CRAVINGS AND ADDICTIONS

Free Yourself from the Struggle of Addictive Behavior with Acceptance and Commitment Therapy

978-1684038336 / US $17.95

newharbingerpublications
1-800-748-6273 / newharbinger.com

(VISA, MC, AMEX / prices subject to change without notice)   Follow Us

Don't miss out on new books from New Harbinger.
Subscribe to our email list at **newharbinger.com/subscribe**

Did you know there are **free tools** you can download for this book?

Free tools are things like **worksheets, guided meditation exercises**, and **more** that will help you get the most out of your book.

You can download free tools for this book—whether you bought or borrowed it, in any format, from any source—from the New Harbinger website. All you need is a NewHarbinger.com account. Just use the URL provided in this book to view the free tools that are available for it. Then, click on the "download" button for the free tool you want, and follow the prompts that appear to log in to your NewHarbinger.com account and download the material.

You can also save the free tools for this book to your **Free Tools Library** so you can access them again anytime, just by logging in to your account! Just look for this button on the book's free tools page.

+ Save this to my free tools library

If you need help accessing or downloading free tools, visit **newharbinger.com/faq** or contact us at **customerservice@newharbinger.com**.